The Healer, The Healing, and The Healed

The Concept Pathology Technique for Perfect Healing

Amanda Plevell

DEDICATION

To all those who pioneer ideas so that we can continue to learn and grow for the healthy benefit of all.

CONTENTS

ACKNOWLEDGMENTS

I acknowledge that as true wisdom is, no wisdom is to one person alone, and no wisdom does not come that first came at some level to someone else. I acknowledge all the healers, intellects, scientists, doctors, that developed all of the strategies that collaborate to make up the Concept Pathology Technique. Your service and contribution to humanity is much appreciated.

How to Use This Book

This book is a working book, meaning it is not going to be read once and then housed on a shelf.

Because it is an essential part of the technique, I would highly recommend taking it to your local office or copy store and have them change the binding to a spiral bound. This way you can flip open to the pages of Categories instead of trying to hold the book open.

I would read through it once or until you understand the jist of the technique, then, begin testing it out on a few subjects. You will develop your flow with practice.

I would secondly create a copy of the categories list so that you can have that near you or on a wall to go down one by one. You might even paste each Illusionary Truth Concept onto vials or tongue depressors for the Healed to hold during testing.

In addition create copies of the worksheet in the back so that as you are in session with a Healed you can easily note which categories where causative and then keep them for reference later.

You have it in you, and you don't need luck. Enjoy!

1 THE CODING OF THE BODY

The body is bio-electrical in nature. Quite simply, for our purposes, it can be compared to a computer system.

The computer, the physical matter of the computer, is the shell, the vessel. Without any code or electricity, it has not use, no purpose, no function.

However, if you send in a programmer, the circuitry stores all of the "code" that the programmer enters. If it wants a space to occur everytime you hit the space bar, it's going to direct the computer to do so by typing a code. Now the computer performs this function without fault, every time and always, without exception. For every function the computer is to perform, the circuit boards are programmed with the appropriate response the programmer wants to elicit.

Even yet, after all of this programming, nothing happens and the computer is without function if it is not attached to a form of energy that runs through the unit, giving it power to function; namely: electricity.

In broad, gross terms, the human body and it's functioning can be seen as such. I do this on purpose. This is not to downplay the amazing essence and spirit that is divine guidance, providence and order. However, as health can be a misunderstood and fearful topic, I merely allow this downplay in order that that fear and misconception can be removed simply by simplifying the processes. We know that of course the life of a human is far more than it's vessel and function. This modality takes that into account and works with the body on every level, physical(corporal), mental, emotional, and spiritual, and other.

So back to our comparison.

Our bodies are merely a vessel built to perform functions that the body carries out. These functions are like that of the "space" action when you hit the space bar on the computer. This coding for every function in the body is stored in every cell of the body, which makes up every tissue, fiber and fluid in the body. While this is physical in nature, this coding is taken in through and affects every other level of the body: mental, emotional, spiritual, and other.

This coding of every cell starts even before conception, but at the very idea within the parents' minds of the possibility, the thought, and even the intention of creating a baby. Truly, it really can start back to the beginning of all life with the first single spark, and follows humanity through all creation and evolutions.

The coding of all things are stored in our cells directing their every action performed outside of and without the help of the conscious mind. Every thought, emotion, feeling, idea, and concept and belief is held in the code of the cells. Every action, behavior, incident, situation, and everything that was learned through them is stored in this code.

3

The DNA and genetic makeup is stored. Everything that was within mom and dad at conception is stored. Every energy that went into this creation is stored. Then as the new being ages and evolves through life, every thing that happens on a moment to moment, daily basis is stored as new directions. However, the new directions, the new codes don't "replace" the old code, unless effort is made for the old code to be absolved, to be deleted, to be negated. Since this was all a subconscious act to begin with, the conscious mind cannot begin to fathom that this is necessary, nor how to go about it. Instead, the conscious mind gets involved with trying to "solve" whatever reason came up for the old code to be absolved, and instead of breaking the energy of the code (cutting off electricity to it) the very act of "thinking" on it creates new synapses, new nerve patterns, new cellular codes and the old code still is not broken, in fact with all of the new pathways these synapses created, there is more "highway" for the codes to travel.

This is where people experience not only a non-healing or non-restoration of balance, but a compounding of seemingly un-solvable symptoms.

Thus, this code is the most important understanding of why the body is performing and functioning the way it is. However, because it is not performed at the conscious level, it is equally hard to recognize what old codes need to be broken.

Second, the energy provided for this code to be performed is equally important. Code cannot be carried out without energy. This energy comes from the thought you give it (good and bad and through your conceptions and beliefs), the energy you put towards it (through action plans, intentions, and attempts at attainment), and the bio-electrical circuitry of the physical being.

2 METHODS COLLABORATION

All of the modalities must be employed to receive stimulus on all levels of the Healed.

1. Body electric stimulus and balance (like chiropractic, electro stimulation therapy, acupuncture, acupressure)

2. Superconscious/subconscious access (like hypnosis)

3. Kinesiology (muscle testing)

And, the people guiding the process:

1. The Healer and the Healed (which is the client)

2. The Protected Space Holding Guide (the one traditionally known as the "healer")

This naming is done on purpose as the client needs to feel like they are not the sick, the ill, the incapable. The body and the essence of the body, and the divine within the body are the only source of healing anyway. This naming puts power back to the only place in this life that can perform healing. We call them the Healed simply because the intention is there that the person's healing is already successful.

The naming of the Guide is important for each term within the name so as to distance the guide from receiving any energies shed from the Healer and the Healed. Simply acknowledging this name is calling in the protective energies.

3

THE CATEGORIES

Complete Categories List

Fundamental (the fundamental 4 are in Bold, the Essential 7 are listed in Italics

Life

Source

People

Healing

Acceptance

Attachment

Roles and Archetypes

Incidentals

Conception

Failure

Incidents or situations

Toxins

Emotions

Body Systems

Colors

Allergies

Foods

Physical Body

Others

Restorative Modalities

Fundamental

Categories

Life Category

Mineral

Carbon

Creation

Generational miasms

Evolution

Each stage and age of existence in any form

Past lives/energies

The first spark of life

Other

Source Category

Self

Someone Else (if this is a hit, go to people category and clear their influence over the Healed)

Source energy (divine, this energy is a cosmic miasm, a healing for the needs of the world, physical or spiritual)

Mainly a physical body issue – go to body systems, then all physical related categories

Mainly a mental body issue – go to thoughts and concepts categories

Mainly a spiritual issue – go to emotions category

Mainly a past life issue – go to life category

Mainly a toxin issue – go to toxins and allergies and body categories

Due to a medical intervention

Due to a post-incident stress – go to incidences category

People Category

Mom

Dad

Spouse or partner

Grandparent

Sibling

Colleague

Authority

Doctor or medical authority

Legal authority

other

Healing Category

Belief

Trust

Faith in self

Faith in the guide

Need for healing

Desire for healing

Willingness to be healed

Willingness to be the healer

Willingness to be healthy

Acceptance of one's own happiness

Other

Acceptance Category –

as a person strongly attaches to their perceptions, concepts, and beliefs, it is necessary to accept the following as underlying in order for healing to happen

Acceptance of Aging

Acceptance of Death

Acceptance of Fear

Acceptance of Guilt

Accdeptance of circumstance

Acceptance of Accountability

Acceptance of Happiness

Acceptance of desire

Acceptance of Joy

Acceptance of Wealth

Acceptance of Poverty

Acceptance of hindering mentalities and mental states

Acceptance of Grief

Acceptance of Loss

Acceptance of non-control

Acceptance of control

Acceptance of thoughts, concepts, beliefs

Acceptance of judgement

Acceptance of non-judgment

Acceptance of all things named and unnamed

Acceptance of self

Acceptance of all other

Attachments category

Attachments to disease

Attachments to diagnosis

Attachments to medical perceived authorities

Attachments to labels

Attachments to concepts, beliefs, ideas, thoughts

Other

Roles and Archetypes category

Label

Role, hat, definition, or any other titled

Victim

Martyr

Lady in distress

Queen/king

Rich man/poor man

Mother

Father

Sister

Brother

Friend

Employee

Coworker

Boss

Other

Incidental

Categories:

Conception Category –

The reason this category is first in the Incidentals and should be tested after the Fundamentals is because of the effects these possible miasmic concepts had on the conception of the Healed. This topic can also later be used for infertility issues

Fear

Fear of pain

Fear of abnormality

Emotions (move to emotion category if yes)

Fear of parenting

Fear of conception

Fertility/infertility issues

Fear of the possibility

Fear of age

Fear of health of the baby

Fear of health of the mother

Fear of success

Fear of failure

Doubt of ability

other

Failure Category

Aborted fetal tissue

Failed idea

Procrastination

Failed business

Failed self

Idea of failure

Other

Incidences or Situations Category

Past illness

 Abuse

Violence

Neglect

Abandonment

Trauma involvement

Legal Crisis

Other

Toxins Category

Bacteria

Virus

Mold

Fungus

Parasites

Chemicals

Inhalants

Metals

Drugs = recreational

Drugs = medical/pharmaceutical

Residues

Personal care products

Toxic thoughts

Dental toxins

Surgical toxins

Illness toxins

All Food Poisons

All Food Toxins

All Ingested Allergies

All Ingested Poisons

All Ingested Toxins

All Inhaled Allergies

All Inhaled Poisons

All Inhaled Toxins

All Injected Allergies

All Injected Poisons

All Injected Toxins

Mercury

Antibiotics

Penicillin

Prescriptions

Supplements

Vaccinations

Preservatives = food

Preservatives = drug

Other

Emotions Category

Anger

Faith

Sadness

Betrayal

Loss

Grief

Happiness

Fear

Joy

Excitement

Love

Pride

Ego

other

Body systems Category

Immune system

Autoimmunity response

Nervous system

    CNS

    Autonomic Nervous System

    Sympathetic Nervous System

    Parasympathetic Nervous System

Digestive system

Circulatory system

Eliminative system

Nervous system

Glandular system

    Prostate

    Adrenals

    Thyroid

    Pineal

    Pituitary

Thymus

Hypothalamus

Muscular system

Colors Category

Red

Orange

Yellow

Green

Blue

Indigo

Violet

Purple

Pink

White

Black

Gray

Brown

All colors

other

Allergies Category =

must be used before all possible causative factor categories, but after spark of life and belief categories

All environmental allergies

All pollens, grasses, trees

Bee

Bee Pollen

I.G.A.

I.G.C.

I.G.E.

I.G.G.

I.G.M.

Histamines

Dog Hair

Dust Mix

Exhaust Mix

Feather Mix

Fish Mix

Insect Mix Macrophage

Macrophage Activating Factor

Macrophage Aggregating Factor

Macrophage Inhibiting Factor

T Lymphoblast

T Lymphocytes

All Airborne Allergies

All Airborne Poisons

All Airborne Toxins

All Contact Allergies

All Contact Poisons

Animal epithelia

Animal hair

Human hair

Human epithelia

All other

Foods Categories

All Canned Food Allergies

All Canned Food Poisons

All Canned Food Toxins

sugar

Egg white (chicken)

Egg yolk (chicken)Gliadin

Gluten

Wheat

Oat

Rice

Grain Mix

Grass Mix

Influenza

All Contact Toxins

M.S.G.

Meat Mix

Milk (cow)

Nightshades

Nut Mix

Soybean

Additives

Preservatives

Bean Mix

Nut mix

Beverages

Fruits

Vegetables

Herbs

spices

Seed Mix

Phenolics

All other

Physical Body Category =

these do not contain biohazard materials, but rather contains only the magnetic charge on which the item can imprint

Your body image

Acceptance of Self

Your Spinal fluid

Your blood waste

Your hormones

Your Skin

Your Sweat

Your Tears

Your Urine

Your Blood

Your Drinking Water

Your Fat

Your Feces

Your Fetus

Your Gravid Uterus

Your Hair

Your Hormones

Your Lubricant

Your Lymph

Menstrual Flow

Your Mucus

Your Myelin

Your Placenta

Your Saliva

Your menstrual fluid

Your Hormones

Your cells

Your tissues

Rejection

Your pathology

Your diagnosis

Biological other

Polarity of cells, tissues, organs

Your Meridians

Your other

Others Category

Unidentified

Unknown

Don't want to know

Fear of knowing

Things missed, hidden, or otherwise unknown

Don't want to identify

Need a modality to identify or restore balance

Need a therapist to identify or restore balance (if this is a hit, clear the belief that the Healed cannot be the Healer, replacing with a belief they can heal themselves)

Restorative Modalities Category

Exercise

Massage

Lymphatic exercise

Aerobic exercise

Weight loss

Spiritual therapies

Concept therapy

Talk therapy

Acupuncture

Chiropractic

Medical

All other modalities – would like to be identified, research further

All other modalities – would not like to be identified

Always add "other" and I do that because of all and any uncertainties and foreign concepts that have yet to be discovered. Also, because all technique is not set in stone, but in perfect balance and order to the Healed's particular need.

Note: the only reason they are named individually and not simply cleared by category is to remove all hooks by acknowledging them directly and also so the Guide can store the information, contemplate their affect and outcome on the Healed, and consciously instruct on further health balance decisions.

4 The Technique

To begin, authority and acceptance of authority must be confirmed. Explain to the Healed their part, that they are responsible for their healing and while they don't physically have to perform anything, the Guide will do that, they have to know they are the only one that can heal.

Name and accept the Client as the "The Protected and Loved healer and the healed".

Name and accept the Guide as the "Protected and Space Holding Guide"

Begin:

1. Ask the Healed to look over a list of all of the categories.

2. Ask them to choose three that stand out as definitely currently problematic for them.

3. Ask them to choose any that stand out as definitely NOT currently problematic for them, the category could not possibly describe them.

This is especially important on the first visit, but is good to ask at each visit, as with each treatment, layers will be cleared, revealing new intuition.

The reason is to remember that the Healed is also the Healer. The healer instinctively knows what is imbalanced within them, but it is on a subconscious level and attention should be paid to what they intuitively believe. Even having the belief, whether physically evidenced or not, is considered an "Illusionary Truth Condition".

Next:

4. Establish polarity by muscle testing positivity and negativity with the Healed's hand palm down on the top of the head, and then the hand palm up on the top of the head. Balance with the hand in palm down position is what is to be established. If it is stronger with palm down position, the Healed is ready. If stronger with hand in palm up position, tap the thymus area and rub the area two inches below the belly button. Test again. The Healed may need some mineral water or a walk around outside if tapping does not establish proper polarity.

5. The Guide accesses the collective subconscious to be able to assist the Healed with identification and treatment, meaning he simply tunes in to the feeling and vibrations around him, making mental note of what he/she picks up.

6. Bring the client to a State of Subconscious Alertness (like hypnosis, where the composite has been formed and the person is willing to cede to all suggestion in the safety of the protected space) by breathing, having them focus on your voice, and "speaking to the subconscious mind, I am here to help even if you don't feel you need it or feel ready for it. It is safe to

release into this protective space all that needs to be made known that the Healed wants to know, is useful for him/her to know, and is necessary for him/her to know. I will be giving you suggestions to accept that will take place of all old and un-useful, even harmful concept to be released, transmuted, and replaced. I want you to perform the new suggestion in place of the old, each and every time the old concept comes up for this person."

Now:

7. Perform the testing lying face up and using the arm to muscle test in the order of the following categories:

Life

Source

Healing

Acceptance

There will not be ability to do all in one session. Try to work on the indicated categories that stood out for the Healed after these initial 4. These Fundamental 4 should be used at the beginning of each treatment.

Test the first 7 categories for need of treatment at each session. Work through clearing these first before moving on to incidental categories. Then work through the incidental categories in the order of whatever the Healed intuitively chose and denied, and then as each category comes up as necessary upon testing.

Work through each category. Once a hit is discovered, the next question should always be "Did this come from the self or someone else?" (you don't always need to know the someone else as this is cleared already. The someone else individual clearing is used when a problem doesn't seem to be clearing up. It could then be coming from someone else and you will need to go to the people category to clear that person.

8. Once the ITC's (the Illusionary Truth concept) categories and individual concepts have been identified, perform the clearing with the healed lying face down. "Across all time space dimensions and realities, release these concepts and all that they may look like, dispersing the energy into the violet flame where it can be transmuted and transformed."

9. Start with the fundamental four, clearing them by name. Before each concept category, tell the Healed, "we are now going to clear _____. What pictures and images do you have springing up surrounding this concept? Then, Use the same guided verbage in #8 and replace "these concepts" with the category name. Now clear any of the Essential 7 that came up before working on the individual concepts.

10. Use a powerful magnet to massage three passes down the spine.

11. Perform a new suggestion, reminding the subconscious that it is to perform the new concept perfectly, deleting and transmuting the old. It is helpful to record these suggestions to continue the care at each session.

12. Bring them back into a now time awareness, calling all parts of their being back.

13. Reflexology or massage on the ears, hands, and feet, and spine while listening to the recorded suggestions is useful to "lock in"

the new suggestive code, as it alerts and engages the neural pathways.

One thing to note: despite of the curiosity involved, I do not put attention or energy on naming or making the Healed aware of what was cleared, as the acknowledgement of it takes away from the healing, rather because of innate victim mentality within the being, this mentality can halt or hinder healing as the person runs the risk of attaching to the "diagnosis" rather than the healing. It is best to simply understand that the necessary healing took place.

14. Give the Healed concepts of affirmation and other modalities for additional wellness to study until the next treatment, giving them the recording is useful.

15. Give any supplements or instructions on beneficial modalities that were discovered

16. Additional coaching as needed by the healed:

Direct nutritional need

Food instructions, what to eat, what not to

 Useful supplementation:

Enzymes

Probiotics

Fish oil

Minerals

Water

Homeopathic imprints - vials of radionically charged mineral water: the body systems, along with any causative factor imprinted within

5 TERMS AND DEFINITIONS

Healed or healer = the person perceiving to need the healing

PSH Guide = the person guiding the healing

Illusionary Truth Condition = the "hits" the yes's, the indicated concepts that are considered to be code that needs breaking, the codes that are no longer working for the Healed's perfect function any longer.

Collective Subconscious = The energy of Oneness that connects all beings.

Violet Flame = known among healing mystics of the dispersion and transformation of all energies back into useful Divine light energy.

Incidental Categories = the categories that indicate any illusionary condition or causative factor that contributed to the problem at hand.

Fundamental Categories = the categories that contain codes that must be cleared before the hooks of Incidentals can be permanently cleared.

Polarity = the state of spin the cells must be in to be in alignment with healing.

Radionically Charged imprints = a healthy person will have certain energy frequencies moving through their body that define health, while an unhealthy person will exhibit other, different energy frequencies that define disorders. Radionically charged water is water prepared for receiving imprints of appropriate frequencies to balance the discordant frequencies of sickness. Radionics uses "frequency" not in its standard meaning but to describe an imputed energy type, which does not correspond to any property of energy in the scientific sense.

State of Subconscious Alertness = The conscious mind steps aside as the subconscious is brought in as the key operating mind.

6 WHO CAN THE TECHNIQUE BE USED WITH?

Animals

Plants

Children

Elderly

All life

In person

Long distance

This technique can and should be used regularly throughout life to delete and transmute energies that can quickly become physical in nature.

Whether or not a disease state is present, the bodies are exposed to multiple levels of energy at a continuous rate. There can only be improvement by using the technique regularly. Worst case scenario is that there will be nothing to clear.

7 FURTHER RESEARCH

For further research of your interest, the roots of the Concept Pathology Technique came from a combination of but not limited to the following methods. I would highly encourage the study of further techniques.

Applied kinesiology

Muscle testing

TBM (Total Body Modification)

NAET (Nambudripad's Allergy Elimination Technique)

Phenolic Therapy

Dr. Thurman Fleet, Concept Therapy

Zone Healing

Radionics http://en.wikipedia.org/wiki/Radionics

Cranio Sacral techniques

Acupuncture, Acupressure

Hypnotherapy

The Emotion Code

Visit Record

Name   Date   Visit Number

Phone   Email

Chief Complaints:

Categories: Notes, supplements,
modalities:

Life	
Source	
People	
Healing	
Acceptance	
Attachment	
Roles and Archetypes	
Incidentals:	
Conception	
Failure	
Incidents or Situations	
Toxins	

Emotions	
Body Systems	
Colors	
Allergies	
Foods	
Physical Body	
Other	
Restorative Modalities	

The Healed, The Healer, and The Healing

The Healed, The Healer, and The Healing

www.ingramcontent.com/pod-product-compliance
Lightning Source LLC
Chambersburg PA
CBHW070948180526
45168CB00003B/1174